LUPUS DIET COOKBOOK: FOR NEWLY DIAGNOSED AND BEGINNERS

Experience Symptoms Relief, Prevent Flares, Reduce Body Inflammation, Enhance Immunity, and Enjoy Easy Weight Loss

Joe Miller, RD

COPYRIGHT PAGE

Copyright © 2024 Joe Miller, RD

Table of Contents

LUPUS AND DIET: AN OVERVIEW

Systemic lupus erythematosus (SLE), colloquially known as lupus, presents itself as a formidable autoimmune disorder with far-reaching impacts affecting a vast number of individuals worldwide. This condition manifests when the immune system, typically tasked with safeguarding the body against harmful invaders, mistakenly turns against healthy cells and tissues. The resultant cascade of inflammation and tissue damage affects diverse areas such as the skin, joints, kidneys, and various organs, casting a wide net of physiological distress.

While the precise triggers of lupus remain elusive, a complex interplay of genetic predisposition, environmental factors, and hormonal influences are implicated in its onset. The intricate web of causation underscores the multifactorial nature of this condition, complicating both its understanding and management.

The relationship between lupus and dietary intake serves as a focal point of ongoing debate and exploration, mirroring similar inquiries into the dietary management of numerous autoimmune disorders. While it's essential to acknowledge that food alone cannot eradicate lupus, judicious dietary choices hold the potential to mitigate its progression and alleviate symptoms. By adopting a holistic approach to nutrition, individuals with lupus can endeavor to quell inflammation, enhance overall well-being, and fortify the immune system.

Central to crafting an effective dietary strategy for lupus management is the identification of potential dietary triggers that may exacerbate symptoms. Certain foods have been implicated in provoking inflammatory responses and precipitating lupus flares, underscoring the importance of personalized dietary adjustments guided by individual responses and sensitivities.

Embracing an anti-inflammatory lupus diet emerges as a popular tactic for taming inflammation and bolstering immune resilience. This dietary approach emphasizes the consumption of antioxidant-rich foods replete with vitamins, minerals, and other bioactive compounds renowned for their anti-inflammatory properties. Fruits, vegetables, whole grains, and healthy fats sourced from nuts and fatty fish feature prominently in this dietary paradigm, offering a nutritional arsenal against the ravages of lupus.

Conversely, certain dietary culprits warrant avoidance for individuals grappling with lupus. Foods rich in purines, such as organ meats and select seafood, may elevate uric acid levels, potentially precipitating gout-like symptoms in susceptible individuals. Likewise, the consumption of saturated and trans fats, pervasive in fried and processed foods, merits restriction due to their deleterious effects on cardiovascular health and propensity to fuel inflammation—a concern heightened among lupus patients.

In addition to specific dietary considerations, some individuals with lupus find relief through exploration of specialized dietary modifications, such as adopting a gluten-free regimen. For certain individuals, particularly those with autoimmune predispositions like lupus, gluten—a protein prevalent in wheat and related grains—may incite gastrointestinal distress and exacerbate inflammation. However, the necessity of gluten avoidance varies among lupus patients and warrants careful deliberation in consultation with healthcare providers.

It's imperative to underscore the individualized nature of dietary interventions for lupus management, necessitating tailored approaches that account for unique physiological nuances and medical histories. Factors such as age, gender, body weight, and comorbidities exert a profound influence on dietary requirements and necessitate nuanced dietary guidance.

This book endeavors to delve into the intricacies of crafting a bespoke lupus diet, encompassing a comprehensive exploration of nutrient relevance, hydration imperatives, meal planning strategies, and adept navigation of social and dining scenarios. Furthermore, it will elucidate potential interactions between lupus medications and specific dietary components or supplements, empowering individuals to make informed decisions for sustained health benefits.

While nutrition undoubtedly plays a pivotal role in the management of lupus, it's imperative to underscore the indispensable role of medical oversight and professional guidance in orchestrating a holistic treatment regimen. Readers are encouraged to engage in open dialogue with healthcare providers before embarking on significant dietary overhauls, especially in the context of preexisting medical conditions like lupus. By embracing a proactive and informed approach to dietary choices, individuals grappling with lupus can seize agency over their health and foster a higher quality of life.

CHAPTER 1
GLUTEN AND LUPUS

The family of grains including wheat, barley, and rye contains a protein called gluten, and over the years, mounting evidence has hinted at a possible relationship between gluten and autoimmune diseases, such as lupus. While our understanding of this connection is still evolving, several studies have suggested that gluten might play a role in triggering or worsening autoimmune reactions in individuals who are sensitive to it.

Understanding how gluten impacts the progression of lupus, a complex autoimmune condition where the immune system erroneously attacks healthy tissues throughout the body, is not always straightforward. The origins of lupus remain elusive, with genetics, environmental factors, and immune system dysfunction believed to contribute to its development.

Recent research has uncovered a potential genetic overlap between lupus and celiac disease, a known autoimmune disorder triggered by gluten. This discovery has prompted further investigation into the potential relationship between celiac disease, gluten sensitivity, and lupus. Gluten sensitivity refers to a condition where individuals experience discomfort after consuming gluten, even without a diagnosis of celiac disease.

Moreover, consumption of gluten has been associated with increased intestinal permeability, colloquially termed "leaky gut." This condition allows undigested gluten molecules and other harmful substances to enter the bloodstream, triggering inflammatory and immunological responses. Such heightened immune activity may exacerbate symptoms or flare-ups in individuals with autoimmune conditions like lupus.

However, it's important to note that not all lupus patients have celiac disease or gluten sensitivity, and not everyone with these conditions may benefit from or require a gluten-free diet. Further clinical research is necessary to establish a definitive link between gluten and lupus, particularly regarding the immediate effects of eliminating gluten from the diet in managing lupus symptoms.

For individuals with lupus who suspect they may have celiac disease or gluten sensitivity, undergoing appropriate testing to confirm the diagnosis is recommended. If gluten sensitivity is confirmed, healthcare providers may recommend a gluten-free diet. However, dietary changes should be made under the guidance of a qualified dietitian or healthcare professional to ensure nutritional balance and overall health.

While preliminary evidence suggests a potential association between gluten and lupus, additional research is warranted to elucidate the precise nature of this relationship and its implications for lupus management. Collaborating closely with healthcare providers is essential for individuals with lupus to determine the most suitable dietary approach based on their unique health circumstances and goals, much like any other dietary modifications.

Grasping the Relationship Between Gluten and Lupus

Ongoing investigations and clinical observations are delving into the intricate relationship between gluten and lupus, shedding light on potential connections and implications within the realm of autoimmune diseases. At the heart of this exploration lies a protein known as gluten, abundantly found in wheat, barley, rye, and their derivatives. Its role as a pivotal player in the onset and progression of certain autoimmune conditions is under scrutiny, with emerging evidence hinting at its possible influence on lupus, an autoimmune disorder characterized by the immune system turning against the body's own tissues and organs.

Comparative analyses between the general populace and individuals grappling with lupus unveil a potentially heightened prevalence of gluten sensitivity among the latter. For those sensitive to gluten, the consumption of gluten-containing foods might incite an inflammatory cascade within their immune systems, manifesting in a spectrum of distressing symptoms such as fatigue, joint discomfort, skin manifestations, and gastrointestinal disturbances. Notably, both gluten sensitivity and lupus share the common denominator of inflammation, prompting speculation among experts that gluten-induced inflammation could exacerbate the symptoms of lupus in susceptible individuals.

Moreover, the concept of "molecular mimicry" emerges as a pivotal consideration in this discourse. This phenomenon posits that certain structural resemblances between protein configurations in gluten and those inherent to the body's tissues might inadvertently trigger the immune system to mount an attack on both, thereby amplifying autoimmune reactivity and inflammation, particularly in individuals genetically predisposed to autoimmune disorders like lupus.

Nevertheless, it's imperative to underscore the nuanced and intricate nature of the gluten-lupus relationship. Not every individual grappling with lupus will necessarily exhibit signs of celiac disease or gluten sensitivity. Furthermore, the precise mechanisms underpinning the interplay between gluten and lupus remain shrouded in complexity and warrant further elucidation through rigorous scientific inquiry.

In light of these complexities, seeking medical evaluation becomes paramount for individuals with lupus harboring suspicions of celiac disease or gluten intolerance. Healthcare providers may recommend specialized blood tests and intestinal biopsies to ascertain the presence or absence of gluten-related conditions. Should gluten sensitivity be identified, the adoption of a gluten-free diet may be advised to alleviate symptoms and potentially mitigate inflammatory responses.

However, navigating a gluten-free diet necessitates meticulous planning under the guidance of healthcare professionals to ensure adequate nutrient intake and avert inadvertent nutritional deficiencies.

Consequently, while a tantalizing connection between gluten sensitivity and lupus emerges, the precise clinical implications and underlying mechanisms demand further elucidation. In navigating decisions pertaining to gluten consumption and its potential impact on lupus management, the indispensable guidance of medical professionals and collaborative efforts with healthcare specialists are indispensable, mirroring the prudent approach advocated for any dietary modifications among individuals grappling with autoimmune disorders.

Controlling Weight and Lupus

Ensuring optimal weight management holds paramount importance for individuals living with Lupus, as the complexities of this autoimmune condition can be exacerbated by fluctuations in weight. Beyond the physical challenges Lupus presents, such as inflammation and medication side effects, the psychological toll of managing weight amidst a chronic illness cannot be overlooked.

The journey towards maintaining a healthy weight for Lupus patients necessitates a multifaceted approach, one that acknowledges the unique needs and circumstances of each individual.

Central to this approach is fostering a collaborative relationship between the patient and their medical support team, comprising professionals like rheumatologists and certified dietitians. Together, they tailor a bespoke weight management strategy, intricately weaving in considerations such as the patient's medical history, current medications, and level of physical activity.

At the heart of this strategy lies the foundational element of nutrition. Embracing a wholesome, well-rounded diet becomes imperative, where whole foods reign supreme. Fruits, vegetables, whole grains, lean proteins, and healthy fats form the cornerstone, offering not only nourishment but also potential anti-inflammatory benefits crucial for mitigating Lupus symptoms. Moreover, the guidance of a registered dietitian becomes invaluable, providing personalized dietary counseling to address any nutrient deficiencies and optimize weight control.

In the realm of portion control, mindfulness takes precedence. Cultivating an awareness of portion sizes empowers individuals to navigate their nutritional intake judiciously, fostering a sense of satiety while preventing overindulgence. Keeping a food journal emerges as a practical tool in this endeavor, facilitating a nuanced understanding of eating habits and calorie consumption patterns.

Complementing dietary measures, regular physical activity emerges as a linchpin in the quest for weight management. However, the dynamic nature of Lupus necessitates a tailored exercise regimen, one that accommodates fluctuations in symptoms and energy levels. Collaborating with a physical therapist or exercise professional ensures the formulation of a safe and effective exercise plan, promoting not only weight loss but also muscle strength and cardiovascular health.

Addressing the often-overlooked aspect of emotional wellbeing, stress management assumes pivotal importance. Stress, a potent trigger for Lupus flares and emotional eating, underscores the need for holistic interventions. Incorporating practices such as deep breathing exercises, mindfulness meditation, and engaging hobbies fosters emotional resilience, thereby fortifying individuals against the adverse effects of stress on weight management.

Furthermore, adequate hydration emerges as a cornerstone of overall health and weight management. Sufficient water intake not only aids in digestion but also curbs appetite, serving as a vital tool in preventing overeating and promoting satiety.

Crucially, setting realistic and achievable weight management goals becomes imperative for long-term success. Opting for gradual, sustainable progress over rapid weight loss safeguards against potential health risks, particularly in the context of chronic conditions like Lupus. By embracing small lifestyle adjustments and fostering a spirit of collaboration with their medical team, individuals with Lupus can chart a course towards enhanced weight control and overall wellbeing.

The Influence of Dietary Choices on Symptoms of Lupus

The connection between the immune system and the digestive tract is profound, exerting significant influence over the manifestations of lupus. In this autoimmune condition, the immune system mistakenly targets healthy tissues, setting off a cascade of inflammation and a diverse array of symptoms impacting various bodily systems and organs. Remarkably, dietary choices can either exacerbate or ameliorate these symptoms, underscoring the pivotal role of nutrition in managing lupus.

Foremost, adopting an anti-inflammatory dietary approach holds promise for individuals grappling with lupus. Given the chronic inflammatory nature of the disease, opting for foods renowned for their anti-inflammatory properties can temper the systemic inflammatory response. Incorporating ample servings of antioxidant-rich fruits, vegetables, and whole grains can quell free radicals and mitigate inflammation. Notably, omega-3 fatty acids found in fatty fish, flaxseeds, and walnuts exhibit potent anti-inflammatory effects, rendering them particularly beneficial for lupus patients.

Moreover, recognizing the substantial presence of the immune system within the gut underscores the imperative of nurturing gut health in those afflicted with lupus. Certain dietary components can disrupt gut integrity, precipitating "leaky gut" syndrome and fostering an overactive immune response. Steering clear of processed foods, refined carbohydrates, and excessive saturated fats is indispensable for preserving gut health. Conversely, prioritizing a diet rich in fiber, probiotics, and prebiotics fosters a favorable gut microbiota environment, bolstering immune function.

Furthermore, discerning specific dietary triggers that may incite lupus flare-ups is paramount. For instance, some individuals with lupus exhibit heightened sensitivity to purine-rich foods, which can elevate uric acid levels and potentially exacerbate joint pain and inflammation. Limiting or avoiding alcohol, seafood, and organ meats can aid in managing these symptoms effectively.

Additionally, maintaining a healthy weight assumes significance in the management of lupus, as excess weight can exacerbate joint strain and inflammation. Engaging in regular physical activity coupled with a balanced, portion-controlled diet facilitates weight management and augments overall well-being.

Lastly, individuals managing lupus often rely on prescription medications to alleviate symptoms, necessitating vigilance regarding potential dietary interactions. Consulting healthcare providers or qualified dietitians is crucial to ensure dietary choices complement medical interventions and do not compromise medication efficacy.

The impact of nutrition on lupus symptoms is multifaceted. Embracing an anti-inflammatory diet, nurturing gut health, and implementing weight-management strategies can mitigate inflammation and enhance overall health. Identifying and circumventing trigger foods can significantly reduce the risk of lupus flare-ups. Collaborating with healthcare professionals to devise personalized, sustainable dietary plans tailored to individual needs and health objectives is indispensable for effectively managing lupus, as with any dietary modifications.

CHAPTER 2
THE ANTI-INFLAMMATORY LUPUS DIET

Crafted with precision and care to cater specifically to individuals battling the challenges of lupus, the Anti-Inflammatory Lupus Diet emerges as a personalized dietary regimen aimed at not only alleviating symptoms but also at addressing the underlying inflammation that characterizes this autoimmune condition.

When the body's immune system turns on itself, as it does in lupus, the repercussions can be far-reaching, resulting in organ damage, discomfort, and pervasive swelling. It's a complex interplay that demands a nuanced approach, and this diet offers a holistic solution by harnessing the power of nutrition.

At its core, the Anti-Inflammatory Lupus Diet centers around the consumption of foods known for their anti-inflammatory properties, fostering a diet rich in fruits, vegetables, whole grains, nuts, seeds, and healthy fats like those found in olive oil and avocados. These dietary staples not only provide essential nutrients but also work synergistically to mitigate inflammatory responses within the body, promoting overall wellness and resilience.

A cornerstone of this dietary approach lies in the incorporation of omega-3 fatty acids, renowned for their potent anti-inflammatory effects. Cold-water fish such as salmon, mackerel, and sardines stand out as exemplary sources of these beneficial fats, while plant-based alternatives like flaxseeds, chia seeds, and walnuts offer viable options for those adhering to a vegetarian or vegan lifestyle.

Conversely, the Anti-Inflammatory Lupus Diet advocates for the avoidance of pro-inflammatory foods, including processed foods, sugary beverages, and items high in saturated and trans fats. Moreover, individuals with lupus are advised to exercise caution with high-purine foods, which can exacerbate joint discomfort by elevating uric acid levels. Foods such as organ meats, seafood, and certain vegetables like asparagus and spinach fall into this category and are best consumed in moderation or avoided altogether.

Furthermore, the potential link between gluten consumption and inflammation cannot be overlooked, prompting some individuals to explore the benefits of a gluten-free approach to manage their symptoms effectively.

Beyond dietary considerations, weight management emerges as a crucial component of the Anti-Inflammatory Lupus Diet. Excess weight not only amplifies inflammation but also imposes undue strain on already compromised joints. By prioritizing nutrient-dense, low-calorie foods and practicing portion control, individuals can work towards achieving and maintaining a healthy weight, thereby alleviating the burden on their immune system and improving overall health outcomes.

Hydration also assumes paramount importance in the management of lupus, as adequate fluid intake supports kidney function and facilitates the elimination of toxins from the body. This is particularly vital for individuals on medication, as certain drugs may increase the risk of dehydration, underscoring the need for vigilant hydration practices.

In addition to mindful eating, the Anti-Inflammatory Lupus Diet underscores the importance of strategic meal planning and preparation. By fostering a proactive approach to dietary choices, individuals can circumvent impulsive decisions that may inadvertently trigger inflammation, thus promoting long-term adherence to the prescribed dietary guidelines.

Moreover, individuals with lupus are encouraged to consult healthcare professionals to assess potential interactions between their medications and specific foods or supplements. Given the intricate interplay between diet and medication efficacy, personalized guidance from qualified professionals is indispensable to ensure optimal health outcomes.

The Anti-Inflammatory Lupus Diet epitomizes a meticulously curated nutritional strategy designed to empower individuals with lupus to proactively manage their condition and enhance their quality of life. By embracing deliberate dietary choices and seeking tailored guidance from healthcare providers, individuals can embark on a journey towards improved health and well-being, transcending the limitations imposed by this challenging autoimmune disorder.

Exploring the Significance of Foods with Anti-Inflammatory Properties

Managing conditions like lupus and other inflammatory diseases often relies heavily on adopting dietary practices aimed at reducing inflammation. In the case of autoimmune disorders such as lupus, where the body's immune system mistakenly attacks healthy tissues, chronic inflammation becomes a persistent issue. This inflammation, a natural response to injury or infection, can significantly exacerbate lupus symptoms, leading to organ damage, fatigue, and joint pain.

In the realm of nutrition, there exists a classification of foods known as anti-inflammatory, which harbor Things Needed capable of mitigating inflammation within the body. Among these beneficial substances are antioxidants, renowned for their ability to scavenge free radicals — unstable molecules known to cause cellular damage and trigger inflammation. Vibrant fruits like berries, leafy greens, and other colorful vegetables stand out as excellent additions to a lupus-friendly diet due to their rich antioxidant content.

Omega-3 fatty acids, found abundantly in fatty fish like salmon, mackerel, and sardines, boast potent anti-inflammatory properties. By inhibiting the production of pro-inflammatory compounds, these fatty acids play a crucial role in reducing overall inflammation levels. Additionally, omega-3s offer a myriad of health benefits, including support for heart health and cognitive function.

Incorporating seeds and nuts, such as walnuts and flaxseeds, into one's diet provides a source of alpha-linolenic acid (ALA), a precursor to EPA and DHA — two other forms of omega-3 fatty acids with further anti-inflammatory effects. Whole grains like brown rice, quinoa, and oats, rich in fiber and phytonutrients, contribute to gut health and help modulate inflammatory responses in the body. Compared to processed carbohydrates, whole grains also promote more stable blood sugar levels, potentially reducing inflammation.

Certain herbs and spices, such as turmeric, ginger, and garlic, contain bioactive compounds renowned for their anti-inflammatory properties. Curcumin, found in turmeric, is particularly well-known for its potent anti-inflammatory effects. Incorporating these herbs and spices into meals can help alleviate signs of inflammation in the body.

While integrating anti-inflammatory foods into one's diet may offer relief from lupus symptoms, it's essential to emphasize that dietary strategies should complement rather than replace medical treatment. A holistic approach to lupus management, including appropriate medication, regular exercise, stress management, and a balanced diet, remains crucial for overall health and well-being. Individuals with lupus should consult with healthcare professionals or qualified dietitians to develop personalized dietary plans tailored to their specific needs and health status.

Crucial Nutritional Elements for Individuals Affected by Lupus

Individuals diagnosed with lupus must pay careful attention to their dietary choices, as a well-balanced diet plays a vital role in bolstering their immune systems, mitigating inflammation, and enhancing overall health. Lupus, a chronic autoimmune disease, demands specific nutrients to support its management effectively.

Omega-3 Fatty Acids stand out as pivotal components in a lupus-friendly diet due to their renowned anti-inflammatory properties. Found abundantly in fatty fish like salmon, mackerel, and sardines, as well as in flaxseeds and chia seeds, these fatty acids hold the potential to alleviate inflammation and alleviate certain lupus symptoms. Moreover, incorporating omega-3s into the dietary regimen may contribute to improved cardiovascular health, a significant concern for lupus patients given their elevated risk of cardiovascular complications.

Antioxidants such as Vitamins C and E, beta-carotene, and selenium play a crucial role in neutralizing harmful free radicals and reducing oxidative stress, a factor implicated in the progression of lupus. Colorful fruits and vegetables like berries, citrus fruits, sweet potatoes, and spinach serve as rich sources of these antioxidants, offering lupus patients a means to combat oxidative damage and support their overall health.

Vitamin D emerges as another essential nutrient for individuals with lupus, vital not only for bone health but also for bolstering the immune system. Due to factors such as limited sun exposure and potential renal impairment, lupus patients often face an increased risk of vitamin D deficiency, making supplementation or careful dietary intake imperative for disease management and bone health preservation.

Calcium intake assumes heightened importance for lupus patients, given their elevated risk of osteoporosis resulting from the disease itself or medications used in its treatment. Sources such as almonds, leafy greens, fortified plant-based milk, and dairy products provide ample calcium to maintain bone density and reduce fracture risk.

Magnesium, crucial for bone health, muscle function, and immune system regulation, may be lacking in some lupus patients due to dietary restrictions or medication side effects. Including magnesium-rich foods like nuts, seeds, whole grains, and leafy greens in the diet can help mitigate potential deficiencies and support overall health.

Dietary fiber plays a vital role in promoting gut health and regulating bowel movements, particularly beneficial for lupus patients prone to digestive issues. Whole grains, fruits, vegetables, legumes, nuts, and legume products serve as excellent sources of fiber, aiding in gastrointestinal health maintenance.

Iron intake is essential for combating anemia, a condition that may arise in lupus patients due to chronic inflammation or medication effects. Incorporating iron-rich foods such as lean meats, beans, lentils, fortified cereals, and leafy greens into the diet can help sustain red blood cell production and alleviate fatigue.

Emphasizing a diversified and nutrient-dense diet comprising a wide array of fruits, vegetables, lean proteins, and whole grains forms the cornerstone of lupus management. Given the individual variations in nutritional requirements, close collaboration with a registered dietitian or healthcare professional is crucial to tailor dietary plans to meet the specific needs and health status of each lupus patient. When combined with appropriate medical care, a balanced diet can significantly contribute to better disease control and overall well-being for those living with lupus.

Dietary Restrictions for Lupus Management

When embarking on a dietary journey tailored for managing lupus, it's imperative to tread with caution, as certain food choices possess the potential to exacerbate symptoms and ignite inflammation within the body. Each individual's triggers may vary, but it's commonly recommended to exercise prudence by limiting or avoiding some of the most notorious culprits.

Primarily, meals abundant in purines merit a discerning eye, as they can precipitate a surge in uric acid levels, consequently fueling joint inflammation. Foods rich in purines, such as liver, kidney, venison, rabbit, and certain types of fish like herring, anchovies, and sardines, warrant a thoughtful approach in lupus management strategies.

Furthermore, the consumption of fried and processed foods, laden with saturated and trans fats, poses a significant concern, as they have been associated with provoking inflammatory responses, potentially exacerbating lupus symptoms. Additionally, processed and packaged food items frequently harbor additives and preservatives, including artificial sweeteners and excessive sodium content, which are notorious for inciting inflammation and are advised to be steered clear of.

For some individuals with lupus, gluten may pose a challenge, as it is found abundantly in wheat, barley, and rye. These individuals may find themselves grappling with gluten sensitivity or experiencing immunological reactions to gluten-containing edibles.

Moreover, excessive intake of sugar-laden beverages and confectioneries may not only lead to weight gain but also fuel inflammation within the body, hence warranting moderation or avoidance.

Lastly, the consumption of alcohol warrants careful consideration, as it may interact unfavorably with certain medications and exacerbate symptoms for some individuals. Thus, its consumption should be limited or abstained from entirely to ensure optimal management of lupus.

In addition to steering clear of these potential trigger foods, it's crucial to cultivate a heightened awareness of one's body and identify any unique sensitivities through Directionss such as maintaining a food journal or seeking guidance from a qualified dietitian. It's paramount to always consult with a healthcare professional before implementing significant dietary modifications, particularly when navigating chronic health conditions like lupus.

Tailoring the diet to accommodate individual needs and preferences can serve as a potent tool in empowering individuals with lupus to effectively manage their condition and enhance overall well-being. By adopting a proactive approach towards dietary choices, individuals can embark on a journey towards improved health outcomes and a better quality of life amidst the challenges posed by lupus.

CHAPTER 3
MEAL PLANNING AND PREPARATION

Crafting an effective dietary regimen tailored specifically for managing lupus entails a comprehensive and strategic approach, centered around meticulous meal planning and meticulous preparation. Individuals grappling with lupus can significantly enhance their symptom management and overall health by proactively organizing their daily meals and snacks well in advance. This proactive stance allows for the seamless integration of a diverse array of anti-inflammatory foods, essential minerals, and potent superfoods into one's dietary repertoire, all while sidestepping potential triggers and inflammatory culprits.

Initiating this journey toward optimal nutrition often begins with the establishment of a weekly meal plan, thoughtfully curated to encompass a spectrum of lean protein sources, wholesome grains, an assortment of vibrant fruits and vegetables, and beneficial sources of healthy fats. By embracing a palette rich in varied colors and flavors, not only does one ensure a nutrient-dense diet, but they also elevate the culinary experience, rendering meals more gratifying and fulfilling.

Integrating immune-boosting fare into these meal plans is paramount for individuals navigating the complexities of lupus. Superfoods like berries, leafy greens, omega-3 fatty acid-rich fatty fish, and almonds can play pivotal roles in mitigating inflammation and fortifying the immune system, thereby offering invaluable support in managing autoimmune conditions like lupus. Moreover, maintaining a well-balanced diet contributes to weight management, thereby alleviating strain on joints and facilitating better control over lupus symptoms.

However, the efficacy of any dietary plan hinges not only on meticulous planning but also on proactive preparation. Streamlining the cooking process and alleviating mealtime stress necessitate prepping components in advance. Whether through batch cooking on weekends or dedicating pockets of time for tasks like vegetable chopping or meat marinating, laying this groundwork significantly simplifies adherence to the lupus diet. By front-loading much of the labor, individuals are better equipped to resist the allure of unhealthy, processed alternatives when dinnertime beckons.

Furthermore, maximizing the utility of leftovers emerges as a savvy strategy within the realm of meal planning. Creating larger portions and strategically freezing leftovers for subsequent meals not only economizes time but also ensures a cache of wholesome options readily available to stave off hunger pangs. Even when navigating external environments such as work or school, maintaining fidelity to dietary goals remains feasible through the preparation of balanced, portable meals.

In tandem with proactive meal preparation, fostering adaptability and openness to adjustments proves indispensable. Recognizing that health needs evolve over time and that certain days may pose greater challenges than others underscores the importance of periodically reviewing and recalibrating the meal plan. This iterative process is instrumental in ensuring sustained progress and long-term success in managing lupus through nutrition.

Ultimately, embracing a conscientious and systematic approach to meal preparation and planning empowers individuals grappling with lupus to reclaim agency over their nutritional intake. By harnessing the potency of a well-balanced, anti-inflammatory diet enriched with immune-boosting superfoods and prepped Things Needed, individuals can mitigate the impact of triggers and inflammation, thereby fostering a greater sense of well-being and contentment amidst the rigors of living with lupus.

Suggestions for Simple and Nourishing Meal Prep

Ensuring a nourishing diet amidst the whirlwind of modern life demands more than just a passing thought. It necessitates a deliberate and strategic approach to meal preparation that not only saves time but also alleviates the stress associated with making healthy choices on the go. By embracing the practice of meticulous meal planning, individuals can pave the way for a consistent intake of nutrient-rich foods, fostering not just physical well-being but also a sense of culinary satisfaction and balance.

The cornerstone of this approach lies in crafting a comprehensive weekly meal plan that caters to both nutritional needs and personal preferences. Embrace a diverse array of nutrient-dense staples, from lean proteins to whole grains, vibrant vegetables, and wholesome fats, ensuring each meal is a celebration of flavor and nourishment. Take into account any dietary restrictions or preferences to tailor the menu to individual tastes, fostering a dining experience that is both fulfilling and enjoyable.

Once the menu is meticulously curated, consider incorporating batch cooking into the routine, particularly during moments of respite such as weekends. This strategic approach involves preparing larger quantities of staple Things Needed like rice, quinoa, grilled chicken, and roasted vegetables, which can then be portioned and stored for easy access throughout the week. By front-loading the cooking process, individuals can significantly reduce the time spent in the kitchen on hectic days, without compromising on the quality or variety of their meals. Investing in high-quality food storage containers further ensures that prepared Things Needed remain fresh and accessible at a moment's notice.

Furthermore, embrace the versatility of certain foods as a means of enhancing efficiency in meal preparation. For instance, a simple roasted chicken can serve as the foundation for a multitude of dishes, from hearty salads to flavorful sandwiches and wraps. Preparing fruits and vegetables in advance by washing and pre-cutting them not only streamlines snack preparation but also facilitates their incorporation into salads and smoothies, promoting a seamless and nutritious culinary experience.

Incorporating time-saving kitchen gadgets such as slow cookers, instant pots, and air fryers can further streamline the cooking process, allowing individuals to enjoy delicious, hands-free meals with minimal effort. By harnessing the power of these tools, one can effortlessly transform basic Things Needed into culinary masterpieces, all while reclaiming valuable time for other pursuits.

To inject an element of excitement and consistency into meal planning, consider implementing themed meal days that cater to various culinary preferences. From "meatless Mondays" spotlighting plant-based delights to "taco Tuesdays" featuring a plethora of filling and topping options, themed meal days add a sense of anticipation and creativity to the weekly menu, ensuring that healthy eating remains both enjoyable and sustainable.

Finally, prioritize hydration as a fundamental aspect of overall well-being. Keep a reusable water bottle within arm's reach throughout the day, encouraging a steady intake of water that not only promotes digestion but also supports optimal health and vitality. By embracing these strategies and incorporating them into their meal preparation routines, individuals can cultivate a sustained and joyful approach to healthy eating, regardless of the demands of modern life. Planning ahead, organizing with purpose, and streamlining the cooking process not only empowers individuals to prioritize their health but also nurtures a deeper appreciation for the nourishing power of food amidst the hustle and bustle of everyday life.

Supplements Advised for Individuals Afflicted with Lupus

In the realm of managing lupus, while the addition of supplements to one's regimen can indeed offer some beneficial support, it is crucial to underscore the indispensable role of a wholesome diet and comprehensive medical care. Supplements ought not to be viewed as substitutes for these fundamental pillars of wellness. Prior to integrating any supplements into your daily routine, it is imperative to engage in a thorough discussion with a qualified medical practitioner.

This is paramount as individual health needs and statuses can vary significantly, necessitating personalized guidance.

Among the spectrum of supplements suggested for individuals grappling with lupus, several hold promise in potentially ameliorating symptoms and enhancing overall well-being. Omega-3 Fatty Acids, abundantly present in fish oil supplements, boast anti-inflammatory properties that may help mitigate the inflammation often associated with lupus. Furthermore, these fatty acids play a pivotal role in maintaining cardiovascular health, a particularly pertinent consideration for lupus patients who may be at an elevated risk of cardiovascular complications.

Another essential supplement deserving of attention in the context of lupus management is Vitamin D. Given the decreased sun exposure and compromised renal function commonly observed in individuals with lupus, there exists a heightened susceptibility to vitamin D deficiency. Supplementation with Vitamin D can serve to bolster the immune system, fortify bone health, and potentially alleviate certain lupus symptoms. It is imperative, however, to exercise caution in dosage management to avert the risk of vitamin D toxicity.

Probiotics represent yet another avenue of supplementation that holds promise for individuals navigating the complexities of lupus. A flourishing gut microbiome is integral to immune system function and overall health. By fostering a healthy gut environment and mitigating inflammation, supplemental probiotics may offer relief from certain symptoms of lupus, as evidenced by emerging research.

Turmeric, enriched with the potent anti-inflammatory compound curcumin, emerges as a compelling supplement for individuals seeking to alleviate lupus-related joint discomfort and inflammation. It is advisable to opt for formulations that enhance curcumin bioavailability, such as those combined with black pepper, to optimize therapeutic efficacy.

Antioxidant vitamins such as Vitamins C and E play a crucial role in combating free radicals and mitigating oxidative stress, both of which are implicated in the pathogenesis of lupus. Supplementation with these vitamins can augment the body's antioxidant defenses, potentially ameliorating lupus symptoms and bolstering overall health.

B-complex vitamins occupy a central position in supporting immune function, neurological health, and energy metabolism. Certain lupus patients may experience deficiencies in these essential vitamins due to specific medications or dietary restrictions, underscoring the importance of supplementation to ensure adequate levels.

Quercetin, a flavonoid renowned for its anti-inflammatory and antioxidant properties, holds promise as a supplemental intervention in the management of lupus. Emerging research suggests that quercetin may attenuate inflammatory responses and alleviate symptoms in autoimmune conditions such as lupus.

Magnesium, a vital mineral involved in myriad metabolic processes, merits attention as a potential supplement for certain lupus patients experiencing low magnesium levels. Given its role in nerve and muscle function, magnesium supplementation may confer symptomatic relief and promote overall well-being.

The inclusion of ginger in one's supplemental regimen presents another avenue for managing lupus-related discomfort and inflammation. Renowned for its anti-inflammatory properties, ginger can be consumed in various forms, including dietary supplements, culinary applications, and herbal teas.

Lastly, Coenzyme Q10 (CoQ10), an antioxidant crucial for cellular energy production, emerges as a compelling supplement for individuals grappling with lupus. Research suggests that CoQ10 supplementation may mitigate symptoms of oxidative stress and contribute to overall health improvement in lupus patients.

LUPUS-FRIENDLY RECIPES

BREAKFAST

Flatbreads with brunch-style eggs

Things Needed

110g self-raising flour, plus extra for dusting

110g atta or plain wholemeal flour

3 tbsp rapeseed oil, plus extra for the bowl and frying

small knob of butter, melted

For the eggs

1 tbsp olive oil

12 cherry tomatoes, halved

4 large eggs

25g grated cheddar

2 tbsp double cream

Directions

STEP 1

Sift the flours and 1 tsp salt into a large bowl. Add 1 tbsp of the oil and 150ml warm water. Bring together into a soft but not too sticky dough (you may need up to 175ml water). If it feels too wet, add some flour. If it's too dry, add water.

STEP 2

Tip onto a floured surface and knead for 4-5 mins, or until smooth. Put the dough in an oiled bowl, cover and leave for 30 mins.

STEP 3

Tip onto a floured surface. Divide into six balls and roll each out into a thin, 18-20cm wide circle using a rolling pin. If you prefer, you can divide again into twelve balls to make smaller flatbreads.

STEP 4

Brush a heavy-based pan with oil and cook one flatbread over a high heat for 1-2 mins on each side, or until golden and starting to puff. Put on a plate and brush with butter. Repeat with the rest of the dough.

STEP 5

Meanwhile, for the eggs, heat the oil in a small non-stick pan and cook the tomatoes briefly until just softened. Season. Crack the eggs into the pan, add the cheese and cream, cover and cook for 2 mins. Remove the lid. Cook until the egg whites are set, then serve from the pan with the flatbreads, making sure the pan has cooled a little first.

Vegan breakfast muffins

Things Needed

150g muesli mix

50g light brown soft sugar

160g plain flour

1 tsp baking powder

250ml sweetened soy milk

1 apple, peeled and grated

2 tbsp grapeseed oil

3 tbsp nut butter (we used almond)

4 tbsp demerara sugar

50g pecans, roughly chilled

Directions

STEP 1

Heat the oven to 200C/180C fan/gas 6. Line a muffin tin with cases. Mix 100g muesli with the light brown sugar, flour and baking powder in a bowl. Combine the milk, apple, oil and 2 tbsp nut butter in a jug, then stir into the dry mixture.

Divide equally between the cases. Mix the remaining muesli with the demerara sugar, remaining nut butter and the pecans, and spoon over the muffins.

STEP 2

Bake for 25-30 mins or until the muffins are risen and golden. Will keep for two to three days in an airtight container or freeze for one month. Refresh in the oven before serving.

Instant berry banana slush

Things Needed

2 ripe bananas

200g frozen berry mix (blackberries, raspberries
and currants)

Directions

STEP 1

Slice the bananas into a bowl and add the frozen
berry mix. Blitz with a stick blender to make a
slushy ice and serve straight away in two glasses
with spoons.

Vegan tomato & mushroom pancakes

Things Needed

140g white self-raising flour

1 tsp soya flour

400ml soya milk

vegetable oil, for frying

For the topping

2 tbsp vegetable oil

250g button mushrooms

250g cherry tomatoes, halved

2 tbsp soya cream or soya milk

large handful pine nuts

snipped chives, to serve

Directions

STEP 1

Sift the flours and a pinch of salt into a blender. Add the soya milk and blend to make a smooth batter.

STEP 2

Heat a little oil in a medium non-stick frying pan until very hot. Pour about 3 tbsp of the batter into the pan and cook over a medium heat until bubbles appear on the surface of the pancake. Flip the pancake over with a palette knife and cook the other side until golden brown. Repeat with the remaining batter, keeping the cooked pancakes warm as you go. You will make about 8.

STEP 3

For the topping, heat the oil in a frying pan. Cook the mushrooms until tender, add the tomatoes and cook for a couple of mins. Pour in the soya cream or milk and pine nuts, then gently cook until combined. Divide the pancakes between 2 plates, then spoon over the tomatoes and mushrooms. Scatter with chives.

Rye bread with almond butter & pink grapefruit segments

Things Needed

4 tbsp almond butter (make your own with the 'goes well with' recipe, right)

1 grapefruit (you will need about 100g flesh)

2 slices rye bread, toasted (optional)

Directions

STEP 1

Toast your rye bread, if you like. Segment the grapefruit and spoon the fruit, along with any juice, into a small bowl.

STEP 2

Spread the almond butter onto the rye bread, and top with the grapefruit, drizzling any juice over the top

Seven-cup muesli

Things Needed

3 cups oats

1 cup mixed nuts including macadamia if possible

½ cup sesame seeds

½ cup sunflower seeds

½ cup raisins

½ cup dried cranberries

1 cup dried ready-to-eat apricots, chopped

To serve

soya or semi-skimmed milk

chopped fresh seasonal fruit, such as pears, banana, pineapple, papya, passion fruit and grapes

Directions

STEP 1

Tip the oats into a large airtight container and add the nuts, seeds, raisins and cranberries. Stir in the apricots.

STEP 2

To serve, spoon a portion into a bowl, pour over the milk and top with chopped fresh fruit.

Smoky rashers & tomatoes on toast

Things Needed

a little rapeseed oil

4 smoked turkey rashers

3 tomatoes, halved

2 slices wholegrain bread

1 tsp English mustard

1 small ripe avocado, stoned, peeled and halved

2 handfuls rocket

Directions

STEP 1

Heat a non-stick pan or griddle and spray or rub with a little oil to lightly grease it. Cook the turkey rashers and tomatoes for a couple of mins each side.

STEP 2

Meanwhile, toast the bread, spread with mustard and squash half an avocado on each. Add the turkey rashers, tomatoes and rocket, and serve hot.

Eggy spelt bread with orange cheese & raspberries

Things Needed

2 medium eggs

2 tbsp orange juice

2 slices spelt bread, halved

50g low-fat cottage cheese

1 tsp orange zest

1 tsp rapeseed oil

50g raspberries

clear honey, to serve (optional)

Directions

STEP 1

Beat the eggs and orange juice in a bowl wide enough to fit the bread in it. Soak the bread in the eggs and juice for 2 mins or so, turning halfway through.

STEP 2

Meanwhile, in a small bowl, mix together the cheese and orange zest. Put the rapeseed oil in a non-stick frying pan over a high heat. When hot, add the eggy bread. Leave to cook for a couple of mins undisturbed, then flip and cook on the other side for another 1-2 mins.

STEP 3

Divide the bread between 2 plates, dollop the cheese on top, followed by the raspberries and honey, if you like

Butternut & cinnamon oats

Things Needed

120g porridge oats

80g raisins

2 tsp ground cinnamon, plus a sprinkling to serve

large chunk butternut squash, peeled and coarsely grated (approx 320g grated weight)

2 x 150ml pots bio yogurt

25g walnuts roughly broken

milk, to serve (optional)

Directions

STEP 1

Tip the oats, raisins and cinnamon into a large bowl and pour over 1 litre cold water. Cover the bowl and leave to soak overnight.

STEP 2

The next morning, tip the contents into a large saucepan and stir in the grated squash. Cook for about 8-10 mins over a medium heat, stirring frequently, until the oats are cooked and the squash is soft. Add a little more water if it's too thick.

STEP 3

Put half of the mixture in the fridge for the next day. Spoon the remainder into bowls, top each portion with 1 pot yogurt and half the nuts. Dust with cinnamon, then serve with a splash of milk.

Spicy Moroccan eggs

Things Needed

2 tsp rapeseed oil

1 large onion, halved and thinly sliced

3 garlic cloves, sliced

1 tbsp rose harissa

1 tsp ground coriander

150ml vegetable stock

400g can chickpea

2 x 400g cans cherry tomatoes

2 courgettes, finely diced

200g bag baby spinach

4 tbsp chopped coriander

4 large eggs

Directions

STEP 1

Heat the oil in a large, deep frying pan, and fry
the onion and garlic for about 8 mins, stirring

every now and then, until starting to turn golden. Add the harissa and ground coriander, stir well, then pour in the stock and chickpeas with their liquid. Cover and simmer for 5 mins, then mash about one-third of the chickpeas to thicken the stock a little.

STEP 2

Tip the tomatoes and courgettes into the pan, and cook gently for 10 mins until the courgettes are tender. Fold in the spinach so that it wilts into the pan.

STEP 3

Stir in the chopped coriander, then make 4 hollows in the mixture and break in the eggs. Cover and cook for 2 mins, then take off the heat and allow to settle for 2 mins before serving.

LUPUS-FRIENDLY LUNCH RECIPES

Herby quinoa, feta & pomegranate salad

Things Needed

300g quinoa

1 red onion, finely chopped

85g raisins or sultana

100g feta cheese, crumbled

200g pomegranate seeds from tub or fruit

85g toasted pine nuts or toasted flaked almonds

small pack each coriander, flat leaf parsley and mint, roughly chopped juice 3 lemon

1 tsp sugar

Directions

STEP 1

Cook the quinoa following pack instructions – it should be tender but with a little bite. Drain well and spread over a platter or wide, shallow bowl to cool quickly and steam dry.

STEP 2

When the quinoa is just about cool stir through all of the remaining Things Neededwith plenty of seasoning.

Cheesy seafood bake

Things Needed

300g medium potatoes (about 3), thinly sliced

2 tbsp milk

40g mature cheddar, finely grated

1 tsp rapeseed oil

1 onion (160g), finely chopped

1 red pepper, deseeded and finely diced (270g)

2 tsp balsamic vinegar

1 tsp vegetable bouillon powder

400g can chopped tomatoes

½ x 30g pack basil, leaves picked and finely chopped

1 garlic clove, finely grated

280g pack skinless cod loins

100g frozen small Atlantic cooked prawns, defrosted

160g broccoli florets

Directions

STEP 1

Boil the potato slices for 10 mins then drain, tip into a bowl and gently mix in the milk and half the cheese. Don't worry if the potatoes break up a little.

STEP 2

Meanwhile, heat the oil in a large frying pan and cook the onion until softened. Stir in the pepper and cook for 5 mins more. Spoon in the balsamic vinegar and bouillon powder, then stir in the tomatoes, basil and garlic. Lay the cod fillets on top, then cover and cook for 6-8 mins until the cod flakes when tested. Heat the grill to high.

STEP 3

Take off the heat, stir in the prawns and tip into a shallow baking dish, breaking up the cod into large chunks. Cover with the potatoes and sprinkle with the remaining cheese. Grill until golden. While it's grilling, steam or boil the broccoli to serve with the bake.

Veggie okonomiyaki

Things Needed

3 large eggs

50g plain flour

50ml milk

4 spring onions, trimmed and sliced

1 pak choi, sliced

200g Savoy cabbage, shredded

1 red chilli, deseeded and finely chopped, plus extra to serve

½ tbsp low-salt soy sauce

½ tbsp rapeseed oil

1 heaped tbsp low-fat mayonnaise

½ lime, juiced

sushi ginger, to serve (optional)

wasabi, to serve (optional)

Directions

STEP 1

Whisk together the eggs, flour and milk until smooth. Add half the spring onions, the pak choi, cabbage, chilli and soy sauce. Heat the oil in a small frying pan and pour in the batter. Cook, covered, over a medium heat for 7-8 mins. Flip the okonomiyaki into a second frying pan, then return it to the heat and cook for a further 7-8 mins until a skewer inserted into it comes out clean.

STEP 2

Mix the mayonnaise and lime juice together in a small bowl. Transfer the okonomiyaki to a plate, then drizzle over the lime mayo and top with the extra chilli and spring onion and the sushi ginger, if using. Serve with the wasabi on the side, if you like.

Giant couscous salad with charred veg & tangy pesto

Things Needed

2-3 raw beetroot (320g), peeled and chopped

3 red onions (320g), cut into wedges

2 green or orange peppers, deseeded and cubed

1 tbsp olive oil

320g cherry tomatoes

200g wholewheat giant couscous

For the pesto

7g fresh coriander, roughly chopped

15g flat-leaf parsley, roughly chopped

1 garlic clove

1 green chilli, deseeded

½ tsp cumin

1 tbsp apple cider vinegar

1 tbsp olive oil

40g pine nuts, lightly toasted

Directions

STEP 1

Heat the oven to 200C/180C fan/gas 6. In a bowl, toss the beetroot, onions and peppers together with the oil, then spread out on a large roasting tray lined with baking paper and roast for 35 mins. Scatter over the cherry tomatoes, then return to the oven for 10 mins more until the tomatoes have softened and the vegetables are tender.

STEP 2

Meanwhile, cook the couscous following pack instructions, then rinse and drain. To make the pesto, put the coriander and half the parsley in a bowl with the garlic, chilli, cumin, vinegar, oil and 25g of the pine nuts. Add 2 tbsp water, then blitz with a hand blender until smooth or use a small food processor.

STEP 3

Toss the roasted veg and chopped parsley through the couscous and pile on the pesto, then scatter with the remaining pine nuts. If you're following the Healthy Diet Plan, serve half of the salad immediately then chill the rest for another day.

Spaghetti puttanesca with red beans & spinach

Things Needed

- 100g wholemeal spaghetti

- 1 large onion, finely chopped

- 1 tbsp rapeseed oil

- 1 red chilli, deseeded and sliced

- 2 garlic cloves, chopped

- 200g cherry tomatoes, halved

- 2 tsp cider vinegar

- 1 tbsp capers

5 Kalamata olives, halved

1 tsp smoked paprika

210g can kidney beans, drained

160g spinach leaves

small handful of chopped parsley

small handful of basil leaves

Directions

STEP 1

Cook the spaghetti in simmering water for 10-12
mins until al dente. Meanwhile, fry the onion in

the oil in a large non-stick frying pan with a lid until tender and turning golden. Stir in the chilli, garlic and cherry tomatoes.

STEP 2

Add the vinegar, capers, olives and paprika with a ladleful of pasta water. Stir in the beans and cook until warmed through.

STEP 3

Add the spinach to the pasta water to wilt, then drain well. Toss with the tomato and bean mixture and the parsley and basil, then pile onto plates or in shallow bowls to serve.

Vegan roast spiced squash salad with tahini dressing

Things Needed

320g diced butternut squash

3 red onions (320g), cut into wedges

2 tbsp rapeseed oil

2 tsp smoked paprika

1 tsp cumin seeds

2 tbsp chopped thyme

125g quinoa

½ x 85g bag kale

2 tbsp pumpkin seeds

2 tbsp tahini

2 tbsp apple cider vinegar

1 garlic clove, finely grated

2 x 400g cans lentils or borlotti beans, very well drained

50g pomegranate seeds

4 generous handfuls of rocket

Directions

STEP 1

Heat the oven to 200C/180C fan/gas 6. Tip the squash and onions onto a large baking sheet and toss with 1 tsp of the oil. Spread out and sprinkle with the paprika, cumin and thyme, then roast for 30 mins.

STEP 2

Meanwhile, cook the quinoa following pack instructions, then drain well (or the base of the salad will be too wet).

STEP 3

Add the kale to the tray of veg, sprinkle over the seeds and return to the oven for 10 mins.

STEP 4

For the dressing, mix the tahini and remaining oil with the vinegar, garlic and 2 tbsp water.

STEP 5

Put the quinoa in a bowl and toss with the lentils or beans. Pile half into a salad bowl and the rest into two lunchboxes or bowls, if you're following the Healthy Diet Plan. Divide the veg on top, then drizzle with the dressing, scatter over the pomegranate seeds and top with the rocket. Chill the other two portions for the next day. Will keep chilled for up to three days.

Spicy vegetable chapati wraps

Things Needed

150g sweet potato, peeled and roughly cubed

200g can peeled plum tomatoes

200g can chickpeas, drained

½ tsp dried chilli flakes

1 tbsp mild curry paste

50g baby spinach leaves

1 tbsp chopped, fresh coriander

2 plain chapatis (Indian flatbreads)

2 tbsp fat-free Greek or natural yogurt

Directions

STEP 1

Cook the sweet potatoes in a pan of boiling water for 10-12 minutes until tender. Meanwhile, put the tomatoes, chickpeas, chilli flakes and curry paste in another pan and simmer gently for about 5 minutes.

STEP 2

Preheat the grill. Drain the sweet potatoes and add to the tomato mixture. Stir in the spinach and cook for a minute until just starting to wilt. Stir in the coriander, season to taste and keep warm.

STEP 3

Sprinkle the chapatis with a little water and grill for 20-30 seconds each side. Spoon on the filling, top with yogurt and fold in half to serve.

Vegan three-bean chilli with potato jackets

Things Needed

2 baking potatoes (about 180g each)

1 tbsp olive oil

1 yellow or orange pepper, deseeded and chopped

2 garlic cloves, finely grated

1 tsp cumin seeds

½ tsp chilli flakes

1 tsp smoked paprika

1 tsp ground coriander

1 tsp dried oregano

400g can chopped tomatoes

2 tsp vegetable bouillon powder

400g can three bean salad (cannellini, flageolet and adzuki), drained handful of coriander, chopped, plus extra leaves to serve

1 small avocado, stoned, halved and chopped or mashed

1 lime, cut into wedges

Directions

STEP 1

Heat the oven to 200C/180C fan/gas 6 and bake the potatoes for 50 mins-1 hr, or until tender.

STEP 2

Meanwhile, heat the oil in a non-stick frying pan and fry the pepper and garlic for a few minutes. Stir in the cumin seeds, chilli flakes and spices, then tip in the tomatoes, bouillon powder and beans. Bring to a simmer, cover and cook for 15 mins, or until reduced to a thick sauce. Stir in the chopped coriander.

STEP 3

Cut a cross into the tops of the baked potatoes and gently press on the sides to open them out. Spoon over the chilli, then top with the avocado and squeeze over some of the lime wedges. Scatter over some coriander leaves and serve with the remaining lime wedges.

Sesame & ginger sushi bowls

Things Needed

25g ginger (choose a straight piece that is quite slim), peeled

4 tbsp raw apple cider vinegar, plus 1 tbsp

200g brown basmati rice

320g frozen edamame beans

1½-2 tbsp tamari

2 avocados, destoned and sliced

1 large carrot, shredded into long matchsticks or coarsely grated

50g cherry tomatoes, halved

¼ cucumber, sliced

2 tsp sesame oil

3 tbsp toasted sesame seeds

Directions

STEP 1

Cut the ginger as thinly as you can to make wafer thin slices or finely shred. Put in a bowl with the 4 tbsp vinegar and 1 tbsp water and massage briefly to soften. Set aside.

STEP 2

Put the rice in a medium pan and add 600ml water. Bring to the boil, cover and simmer on a low heat for 15 mins. Tip in the edamame beans, but don't stir them in, then cover and cook for 7 mins more. The rice should be tender and have absorbed all the water.

STEP 3

Skim the beans off the rice and set aside. Tip the 1 tbsp of vinegar and ½ tbsp tamari into the rice, and stir well. Spoon onto a plate and spread out to cool quickly. Once cool, spoon into four bowls or lunchboxes. Top with the avocado, carrot, beans, tomatoes and cucumber.

STEP 4

Spoon the ginger from the vinegar and scatter on top. Add the remaining tamari and sesame oil to the vinegar. Spoon over the sushi bowl and scatter with the seeds. Will keep in the fridge for two days.

Feta & clementine lunch bowl

Things Needed

1 red onion, halved and thinly sliced

1 lemon, zested and juiced

2 clementines, 1 zested, flesh sliced

2 garlic cloves, chopped

400g can green lentils, drained

1 tbsp balsamic vinegar

1 ½ tbsp rapeseed oil

1 red pepper, quartered and sliced

60g feta, crumbled

small handful mint, chopped

4 walnut halves, chopped

Directions

STEP 1

Mix the onion with the lemon juice, lemon and clementine zest and garlic.

STEP 2

Tip the lentils into two bowls or lunchboxes and drizzle over the balsamic and 1 tbsp oil. Heat the remaining oil in a large non-stick wok, add the pepper and stir-fry for 3 mins. Tip in half the onion and cook until tender. Pile on top of the lentils, then mix the clementines, remaining onions, feta, mint and walnut pieces.

Mango salad with avocado and black beans

Things Needed

1 lime, zested and juiced

1 small mango, stoned, peeled and chopped

1 small avocado, stoned, peeled and chopped

100g cherry tomatoes, halved

1 red chilli, deseeded and chopped

1 red onion, chopped

½ small pack coriander, chopped

400g can black beans, drained and rinsed

Directions

STEP 1

Put the lime zest and juice, mango, avocado, tomatoes, chilli and onion in a bowl, stir through the coriander and beans.

LUPUS-FRIENDLY DINNER RECIPES

Braised beef with ginger

Things Needed

rapeseed oil

1 ¼kg beef shin or brisket, cut into very large chunks

2 onions

50g ginger

3 garlic cloves

small bunch coriander

2 tsp Chinese five-spice powder

6 whole star anise

1 tsp black peppercorn

100g dark brown muscovado sugar

50ml light soy sauce

50ml dark soy sauce

2 tbsp tomato purée

beef stock

To serve

thumb-sized chunk ginger, shredded into matchsticks

1 tbsp vegetable or sunflower oil

cooked jasmine rice

Directions

STEP 1

Heat a little of the oil in a large flameproof dish. Add the beef chunks, in batches, and fry until browned. When each batch is browned, transfer the beef to another dish. Very roughly chop the onions, ginger, garlic and coriander stalks. Put in a food processor and whizz to a paste.

STEP 2

Wipe any oil out of the dish you browned the beef in. Add the paste with a good splash of water and gently fry, scraping up any beef bits, until the paste is fragrant and softened (add more water if the paste sticks). Stir in the five-spice, star anise and peppercorns, cook for 1 min, then add the sugar, soy sauces and tomato purée. Return the beef and any juices to the dish, then stir in enough stock to just about cover. Bring to a gentle simmer. Heat oven to 160C/140C fan/gas 3. Cover the dish, put in the oven and cook for 21/2 hrs until the beef is really tender.

STEP 3

Lift the beef out of the sauce into a dish, to keep warm. Boil the sauce until reduced by about half and thickened. Meanwhile, fry the ginger in the oil until golden and crispy. Return the beef to the sauce. serve the beef spooned over rice and scattered with the crispy ginger.

Chicken parmesan

Things Needed

2 large, skinless chicken breasts, halved through the middle

2 eggs, beaten

75g breadcrumb

75g parmesan, grated

1 tbsp olive oil

2 garlic cloves, crushed

half a 690ml jar passata

1 tsp caster sugar

1 tsp dried oregano

half a 125g ball light mozzarella, torn

Directions

STEP 1

Halve 2 large skinless chicken breasts through the middle then place the 4 pieces between cling film sheets and bash out with a rolling pin until they are the thickness of a £1 coin.

STEP 2

Dip in 2 beaten eggs, then 75g breadcrumbs, mixed with half of the 75g grated parmesan. Set aside on a plate in the fridge while you make the sauce.

STEP 3

Heat 1 tbsp olive oil and cook 2 crushed garlic cloves for 1 min, then tip in half a 690ml jar passata, 1 tsp caster sugar and 1 tsp dried oregano. Season and simmer for 5-10 mins.

STEP 4

Heat grill to High and cook the chicken for 5 mins each side, then remove.

STEP 5

Pour the tomato sauce into a shallow ovenproof dish and top with the chicken.

STEP 6

Scatter over torn pieces of half a 125g ball light mozzarella, and the remaining grated parmesan and grill for 3-4 mins until the cheese has melted and the sauce is bubbling.

STEP 7

Serve with vegetables or salad and some pasta or potatoes, if you like.

Cheat's beetroot biriyani

Things Needed

3 large (500g unprepped), raw beetroot, peeled and cut into 2cm cubes

2 tbsp rapeseed oil

1 large onion, finely sliced

thumb-sized piece of ginger, grated

2 small garlic cloves, crushed

1 bay leaf

4 cardamom pods

2 tsp turmeric

2 tbsp garam masala

250g basmati rice, rinsed

500ml low-salt veg stock

100ml fat-free yogurt

small bunch of coriander

your favourite chutney or pickle, to serve (optional)

Directions

STEP 1

Heat the oven to 200C/180C fan/gas 6. Toss the beetroot with half the oil and some seasoning, then tip into a roasting dish and cook for 25-30 mins, tossing halfway through, until tender.

STEP 2

Meanwhile, heat the remaining oil in a large, shallow casserole dish or ovenproof frying pan. Fry the onion over a medium heat for 10 mins until golden. Add the ginger and half the garlic, and cook for 1 min. Stir through the bay, cardamom pods, turmeric and garam masala, then cook for 2 mins. Stir in the rice and beetroot, then season. Pour in the stock and bring to the boil.

STEP 3

Put in the oven, uncovered, and cook for 20-25 mins until the rice is cooked through. Give it a stir when it's out of the oven.

STEP 4

Put the yogurt, coriander and remaining garlic in a food processor and whizz until smooth. Season to taste. Serve the biriyani with the coriander yogurt and pickle.

Braised pork with plums

Things Needed

about 1.6kg/3lb 8oz pork shoulder

5 tbsp rice wine

5 tbsp light soy sauce for flavour, 1 tbsp dark for colour

generous thumb-size piece fresh root ginger

5 garlic cloves

1 red chilli, deseeded and finely chopped

2 tbsp vegetable oil

bunch spring onions, finely sliced

2 star anise

1 ½ tsp five-spice powder

1 cinnamon stick

2 tbsp sugar, any type

1 tbsp tomato purée

500ml chicken stock

6 ripe plums, halved and stoned

Directions

STEP 1

Cut the pork into big pieces about the length of your thumb and twice as wide. Put into a bowl or food bag, and add the wine, soy sauces, half the ginger, half the garlic and half the chilli. Marinate for at least 1 hr or up to 24 hrs.

STEP 2

Heat oven to 160C/140C fan/gas 3, then heat the oil in a large casserole. Tip in half the spring onions, remaining ginger and garlic, the star anise, five-spice powder and cinnamon. Fry gently until fragrant and soft. Stir in the sugar, turn up the heat, then lift the pork from the marinade and turn in the oniony mix for about 3 mins until the meat is just sealed but not browned. Tip in the marinade, tomato purée and stock, give it a stir, cover, then braise in the oven for 2 hrs.

STEP 3

After the first hr is up, add the plums to the pan. Take the lid off and carry on the cooking, uncovered. The meat should be completely tender, turning golden brown where it breaks the surface of the sauce. Spoon off any excess fat from the surface, then scoop the meat and plums carefully from the pan with a slotted spoon. Turn up the heat and boil the sauce for 5-10 mins until reduced and slightly syrupy. Return everything to the pan, gently warm through, then scatter the rest of the spring onions over the top to serve.

One-pot paneer curry pie

Things Needed

2 tbsp vegetable oil

440g paneer, cut into 2cm cubes

4 tbsp ghee or butter

2 large onions, finely sliced

2 large garlic cloves, crushed

thumb-sized piece of ginger, finely grated

½ tsp hot chilli powder

2 tsp ground cumin

2 tsp fenugreek seeds

1½ tbsp garam masala

2 x 400g cans chopped tomatoes

1 tbsp caster sugar

300g potato, peeled and cut into 2cm cubes

150g spinach

150g frozen peas

100ml double cream

2 tbsp cashew nut butter

plain flour, for dusting

320g sheet all-butter puff pastry

2 large eggs, 1 whole, 1 yolk only, lightly beaten together (freeze the leftover egg white for another recipe)

2 tsp nigella seeds

pilau rice or green veg, to serve

Directions

STEP 1

Heat the oil over a medium heat in a shallow flameproof casserole dish roughly 30cm wide. Add the paneer and fry for 5 mins, turning with tongs until each side is golden. Remove from the pan and set aside on a plate lined with kitchen paper.

STEP 2

Heat the ghee or butter in the same dish over a medium-low heat, then add the onions and a big pinch of salt. Fry for 15 mins, or until softened and caramelised. Stir in the garlic and ginger, cook for 1 min, then tip in the spices and fry for a further 2 mins. Scrape the spiced onions into a food processor or blender along with the tomatoes and blitz until smooth. Pour back into the pan with 1½ cans of water, then stir through the sugar and potatoes. Bring to the boil, lower to a simmer, then cover and cook, stirring occasionally, for 20-25 mins or until the potato is just tender.

STEP 3

Add the spinach and peas, and cook for 5 mins. Stir in the cream and cashew butter, then return the paneer to the pan and season to taste. Remove from the heat and set aside to cool completely.

STEP 4

Heat the oven to 220C/200C fan/gas 8. On a lightly floured surface, roll the pastry out to just bigger than your casserole dish. Cut a thin strip off each side and fix these around the edge of the casserole. Roll the pastry sheet over the top and press the edges with a fork to seal, and tuck in any overhang. Brush with the egg, sprinkle with the nigella seeds and bake for 30-35 mins or until deep golden brown. Leave to rest for 15 mins before serving with pilau rice or green veg.

Doner kebab

Things Needed

500g lamb mince

1 small onion, coarsely grated

4 garlic cloves, minced or finely grated

100g fresh breadcrumbs

2 tsp ground cumin

2 tsp ground coriander

1 tsp dried oregano

¼ tsp smoked paprika

sunflower oil for oiling

To serve

pitta breads, shredded red or white cabbage, sliced onion, chopped tomatoes, pickled chillies, chilli sauce (see recipe below), garlic sauce (see recipe below), tahini

Directions

STEP 1

Heat the oven to 200C/180C fan/gas 6. Tip all the Things Neededexcept the oil into a food processor with a large pinch of salt and lots of ground pepper. Pulse until everything is combined and chopped together. You can also just squish everything together in a bowl but this will give you a looser finish.

STEP 2

Oil a large sheet of foil, tip the meat mix in the middle and mould to a very thick sausage, roughly the shape of an aubergine. Roll up the foil tightly, twisting up the ends to create a Christmas cracker shape.

STEP 3

Lay on a shallow roasting tin and roast in the oven for 35-40 mins, turning occasionally, or until a digital cooking thermometer reads 75C when pierced in the middle. Leave the kebab to cool a little, then unwrap the foil. Place back on the tray and brown under the grill or with a blowtorch.

STEP 4

Place on a board and carve into thin slices. For full doner mode, you can hold the kebab up with a roasting fork or metal skewer and carve. Serve with warm pitta bread and any of the other accompaniments, including our chilli sauce and garlic yogurt sauce.

Roasted carrot & whipped feta tart

Things Needed

large bunch of carrots with tops (about 800g)

2 tsp olive oil

1 tsp za'atar

2 tsp honey

125-150ml extra virgin olive oil

2 garlic cloves, roughly chopped

50g walnuts, roughly chopped

40g grated parmesan or vegetarian hard cheese

25g parsley, roughly chopped, plus whole leaves to serve

200g feta drained and crumbled (vegetarian, if needed)

150g Greek yogurt

1 lemon, zested

500g block puff pastry

1 egg, beaten

Directions

STEP 1

Heat the oven to 200C/180C fan/gas 6. Trim off the carrot tops, discarding any tough stems, then set aside. Halve the carrots lengthways, tip into a roasting tin and toss with the olive oil and some seasoning. Roast for 25-30 mins until tender and golden, stirring once or twice to ensure they don't stick. Stir in the za'atar and honey, and set aside.

STEP 2

Meanwhile, tip the reserved carrot tops and extra virgin olive oil into a food processor. Season and blitz, scraping down the sides occasionally until finely chopped. Add the garlic, walnuts, parmesan and parsley, and pulse until combined. Pour in another splash of olive oil, if needed. Transfer to a bowl and season to taste. Clean out the food processor, then tip in the feta, yogurt, most of the lemon zest and some seasoning. Blitz until smooth and creamy.

STEP 3

Put a large baking tray in the oven to heat up. Roll the pastry out on a sheet of baking parchment into a roughly 40 x 30cm rectangle. Gently score a 2cm border around the edge using a sharp knife. Brush the beaten egg all over the pastry and sprinkle a large pinch of sea salt around the border. Carefully slide the pastry onto the hot baking tray using the parchment to help you, and bake for 15-20 mins until golden and puffed up. Remove from the oven and gently press the middle down using the back of a metal spoon. Cool for 5-10 mins, then spread the whipped feta over the middle and arrange the roasted carrots on top. Drizzle over the pesto, scatter over the parsley and the remaining lemon zest, and cut into slices to serve.

Aromatic prawn & cashew curry

Things Needed

1 onion, chopped

thumb-sized piece ginger, peeled and roughly chopped

4 garlic cloves, peeled

2 green chillies, seeds removed

small bunch coriander, stalks roughly chopped, leaves picked

1 tbsp butter or ghee

1 tbsp sunflower oil

2 tbsp garam masala

150g bag unsalted cashew

400g can chopped tomato

400ml chicken stock

400g raw king prawn

150ml pot natural yogurt

50ml double cream

rice and Indian breads, to serve

Directions

STEP 1

Put the onion, ginger, garlic, chillies and coriander stalks in a small food processor, or pestle and mortar, and mix to a paste. Meanwhile, heat the butter or ghee and oil in a large pan. Add the paste to the pan and stir-fry for 5 mins to soften. Add the garam masala and cook for a further 2 mins until aromatic.

STEP 2

Meanwhile, toast the cashew nuts in a small pan until golden. Tip half into the food processor and blend until finely ground. Set aside the remaining cashews.

STEP 3

Add the blended cashews, the tomatoes and the chicken stock to the pan. Season and bring to a boil, then lower the heat and simmer, covered with a lid, for 45 mins. Add the prawns and cook for a further 2-3 mins until they turn pink, then add the yogurt and double cream and stir well. Scatter with the coriander leaves and the remaining cashew nuts, and serve with rice and naan bread.

Kidney bean curry

Things Needed

1 tbsp vegetable oil

1 onion, finely chopped

2 garlic cloves, finely chopped

thumb-sized piece of ginger, peeled and finely chopped

1 small pack coriander, stalks finely chopped, leaves roughly shredded

1 tsp ground cumin

1 tsp ground paprika

2 tsp garam masala

400g can chopped tomatoes

400g can kidney beans, in water

cooked basmati rice, to serve

Directions

STEP 1

Heat the oil in a large frying pan over a low-medium heat. Add the onion and a pinch of salt and cook slowly, stirring occasionally, until softened and just starting to colour. Add the garlic, ginger and coriander stalks and cook for a further 2 mins, until fragrant.

STEP 2

Add the spices to the pan and cook for another 1 min, by which point everything should smell aromatic. Tip in the chopped tomatoes and kidney beans in their water, then bring to the boil.

STEP 3

Turn down the heat and simmer for 15 mins until the curry is nice and thick. Season to taste, then serve with the basmati rice and the coriander leaves.

Ravioli lasagna

Things Needed

1 tbsp vegetable oil

1 onion, finely chopped

2 garlic cloves, finely chopped

thumb-sized piece of ginger, peeled and finely chopped

1 small pack coriander, stalks finely chopped, leaves roughly shredded

1 tsp ground cumin

1 tsp ground paprika

2 tsp garam masala

400g can chopped tomatoes

400g can kidney beans, in water

cooked basmati rice, to serve

Directions

STEP 1

Heat the oil in a large frying pan over a low-medium heat. Add the onion and a pinch of salt and cook slowly, stirring occasionally, until softened and just starting to colour. Add the garlic, ginger and coriander stalks and cook for a further 2 mins, until fragrant.

STEP 2

Add the spices to the pan and cook for another 1 min, by which point everything should smell aromatic. Tip in the chopped tomatoes and kidney beans in their water, then bring to the boil.

STEP 3

Turn down the heat and simmer for 15 mins until the curry is nice and thick. Season to taste, then serve with the basmati rice and the coriander leaves.

LUPUS-FRIENDLY DESSERT RECIPES

Carrot patch cake

Things Needed

175ml vegetable oil, plus extra for the tin

75g natural yogurt

3 large eggs

1 tsp vanilla extract

200g self-raising flour

250g light muscovado sugar

2 tsp ground cinnamon

¼ fresh nutmeg, finely grated

200g carrots (about three), grated

100g sultanas or raisins

100g pistachios, finely chopped (or slivered if you can get them)

For the icing

100g slightly salted butter, softened

200g icing sugar

100g full-fat cream cheese

100g fondant icing or marzipan

orange food colouring

Directions

STEP 1

Heat oven to 180C/160C fan/gas 4. Oil and line a 900g loaf tin with baking parchment. Whisk the oil, yogurt, eggs and vanilla in a jug. Mix the flour, sugar, cinnamon and nutmeg with a good pinch of salt in a bowl. Squeeze any lumps of sugar through your fingers, shaking the bowl a few times to bring the lumps to the surface.

STEP 2

Add the wet Things Neededto the dry, along with the carrots, raisins and half the pistachios. Mix well to combine, then scrape into the tin. Bake for 1 hr 10 mins or until a skewer inserted into the centre of the cake comes out clean. If any wet mixture clings to the skewer, return to the oven for 5 mins, then check again. Leave to cool in the tin.

STEP 3

To make the icing, beat the butter and sugar together until smooth. Add half the cream cheese and beat again, then add the rest (adding it bit by bit prevents the icing from splitting). Remove the cake from the tin and spread the icing thickly on top. Scatter with some of the remaining pistachios. Dye the fondant or marzipan orange by kneading in a drop of food colouring. Roll into little carrot shapes, then use a skewer to make indentations and poke a few pistachios in to look like fronds. Top the cake with the carrots, then serve. Will keep in the fridge for up to five days (eat at room temperature).

Champagne & raspberry possets

Things Needed

140g frozen raspberries, defrosted

2 tbsp champagne (buy a mini bottle and treat yourself to a glass while you prepare dinner!)

200ml double cream

4 tbsp golden caster sugar

2 tsp freeze-dried raspberry pieces

shortbread biscuits, to serve

Directions

STEP 1

Put the raspberries and Champagne in a mini food processor or blender (or use a jug and a hand blender). Whizz until the purée is as smooth as you can get it, then use a wooden spoon or spatula to push as much of it through a sieve as you can. Discard the seeds left behind.

STEP 2

Put the cream and sugar in a saucepan and warm gently until the sugar melts. Increase the heat until just boiling, then boil vigorously for 2 1/2 mins, stirring constantly. Turn off the heat and stir in the raspberry-Champagne purée. Cool for 15 mins before dividing between 2 small pots or glasses. Chill for 30 mins, then sprinkle over the freeze-dried raspberry pieces and chill for at least 2 hrs more until set (or overnight if you're making ahead).

STEP 3

To serve, remove the possets from the fridge and add some shortbread biscuits (shop-bought or find shortbread recipes here on bbcgoodfood.com).

Frozen tropical fruit yogurt

Things Needed

480g frozen tropical fruit mix

170g Greek yogurt

2 tbsp maple syrup or honey

200g diced tropical fruit and passion fruit seeds, to serve

Directions

STEP 1

Put everything except the fresh fruit in a food processor and blend. Scoop straight into bowls, or tip into a container and freeze if you want to serve it later. Serve with the fresh tropical fruit and spoon over the passion fruit seeds.

Bourbon biscuits

Things Needed

125g soft unsalted butter

125g golden caster sugar, plus extra for sprinkling

2 tbsp golden syrup

1 large egg, lightly beaten

250g plain flour, plus extra for dusting

50g cocoa powder

1 tsp baking powder

For the filling

150g unsalted butter, softened

360g icing sugar, sifted

4 tbsp cocoa powder

pink food colouring

Directions

STEP 1

Beat the butter and sugar together until creamy, then mix in the rest of the Things Needed. Add a splash of milk if the mixture looks a bit dry – it should come together as a dough.

STEP 2

Line three baking sheets, dust lightly with flour, then roll and pat one-third of the dough out to the thickness of a £1 coin on each. Cover and freeze for 15 mins.

STEP 3

Heat oven to 180C/160C fan/gas 4. Slide the dough off the trays and put a new piece of parchment on each. Trim the edges of the dough to straighten, then cut into rectangles, roughly 6 x 3cm. Lift each one carefully onto the tray, leaving some space between them as they'll expand. Bourbons usually have a pricked pattern, so use a cocktail stick to do this if you want (not too many or they'll break up). Put the dough back in the freezer if it gets too soft.

STEP 4

Bake for 8-10 mins, then leave to cool on the sheet as the biscuits will be soft when they're hot. Sprinkle over some sugar. Will keep for a week in an airtight container.

STEP 5

Meanwhile, make the filling. Beat the butter and icing sugar together, then divide the mixture into three. Add the cocoa to one lot, a dot of pink colour to another, and leave the last one plain (add a little more icing sugar if you need to). Spoon each into a piping bag or a sandwich bag with the corner snipped off.

STEP 6

When the biscuits have cooled completely, pipe the icings onto half of them, then sandwich together with the other halves. Leave to set.

Easy chocolate chip cookies

Things Needed

120g butter, softened

75g light brown sugar

75g golden caster sugar

1 medium egg

1 tsp vanilla extract

180g plain flour

½ tsp bicarbonate of soda

150g dark chocolate, cut into chunks

Directions

STEP 1

Heat oven to 180C/160C fan/gas 4 and line two baking sheets with parchment. Cream the butter and sugars together until very light and fluffy, then beat in the egg and vanilla. Once combined, stir in the flour, bicarb, chocolate and ¼ tsp salt.

STEP 2

Scoop 10 large tbsps of the mixture onto the trays, leaving enough space between each to allow for spreading. Bake for 10-12 mins or until firm at the edges but still soft in the middle – they will harden a little as they cool. Leave to cool on the tray for a few mins before eating warm, or transfer to a wire rack to cool completely. Will keep for three days in an airtight container.

Vegan cookies & cream cake

Things Needed

150ml sunflower oil, plus extra for the tin

200ml dairy-free milk (we used oat milk)

1 ½ tsp white wine vinegar

1 tsp vanilla extract

120g dairy-free yogurt (we used coconut yogurt)

225g light brown soft sugar

200g self-raising flour

70g cocoa powder

1 tsp baking powder

½ tsp bicarbonate of soda

For the icing and decoration

150g crème-filled chocolate sandwich cookies

150g vegan spread

1 tsp vanilla extract

275g icing sugar

Directions

STEP 1

Oil a 20 x 20cm baking tin and line the base and sides with baking parchment. Heat the oven to 180C/ 160C fan/gas 4. Combine the oil, milk, vinegar, vanilla and yogurt in a jug. Mix the sugar, flour, cocoa powder, baking powder, bicarb and a pinch of salt together in a bowl.

STEP 2

Pour the wet Things Neededinto the dry and mix until there are no pockets of flour remaining. Tip the mixture into prepared tin and level the surface with a spatula. Bake for 35 mins, or until a skewer inserted into the middle of the cake comes out clean. If any wet cake mixture clings to the skewer, return the cake to the oven for another 5 mins, then check again. Remove from the oven and leave to cool completely in the tin.

STEP 3

Set half of the cookies aside for decorating later. Bash the rest with the end of a rolling pin or blitz in a food processor to chunky rubble. Beat the spread, vanilla and icing sugar together using an electric whisk until fluffy, then gently fold in the crushed cookies until combined.

STEP 4

Put the cake on a board. Spread over the icing. Halve or crumble the rest of the cookies and use these to decorate. Cut into squares. Will keep in an airtight container for four days.

Devil's food cake

Things Needed

200g unsalted butter, plus extra for the tins

200g dark chocolate, chopped

250g plain flour

50g rye or spelt flour (or use 50g plain flour)

50g cocoa, sifted, plus extra for dusting

2 tsp baking powder

1 tsp bicarbonate of soda

400g light muscovado sugar

300ml natural yogurt

150ml espresso or strong coffee

2 tsp vanilla extract

3 eggs

For the icing

300g dark chocolate, chopped into small pieces

400g unsalted butter, softened

300g icing sugar, sifted

50g cocoa powder

100ml milk

Directions

STEP 1

Heat the oven to 180C/160C fan/gas 4. Butter the base of two 20cm springform cake tins and line with baking parchment. Melt the butter and chocolate in a heatproof bowl over a pan of simmering water (make sure the base of the bowl doesn't touch the water), or do this in the microwave in 10-second bursts. Set aside. Put the flours, cocoa powder, baking powder, bicarbonate of soda, sugar and ½ tsp salt in a bowl, and mix well. If there are any lumps in the sugar, squeeze these through your fingers to break them up.

STEP 2

Put the yogurt, coffee, and vanilla in a jug, and whisk in the eggs until smooth. Pour the wet Things Needed, along with the melted chocolate mixture, into the dry Things Needed. Fold everything together until well combined.

STEP 3

Divide the cake batter evenly between the two tins, and bake for 30 mins, or until risen and a skewer inserted into the centres comes out clean. Leave to cool in the tins for 10 mins, then turn out onto a wire rack, peel off the baking parchment and leave to cool completely. Once cooled, the cakes will keep, well wrapped, for up to three days.

STEP 4

To make the icing, melt the chocolate as you did in step 1. Cool slightly. Put the butter, icing sugar and cocoa in a large bowl and mash together, then beat with an electric whisk until smooth. Add the melted chocolate and milk, then mix until smooth.

STEP 5

Split the cakes in half through the equator using a bread knife. Secure one layer to a board or plate using a little icing. Spread over a layer of icing, sprinkle over a little sea salt, then sandwich with another cake layer. Repeat until about half the icing and all the remaining cake layers have been used, ensuring the final layer is flat-side up. Spread the remaining icing all over the cake using a palette knife to smooth it, or swipe upwards around the side for texture. Dust with cocoa powder and sprinkle with sea salt flakes. Will keep covered for up to four days.

Biscuity lime pie

Things Needed

300g pack ginger nut biscuit

100g butter, melted

3 egg yolks

50g golden caster sugar

zest and juice 4 lime, plus thin lime slices (optional) to serve

zest juice 1 lemon

397g sweetened condensed milk

Directions

STEP 1

Heat oven to 180C/fan 160C/gas 4. Tip the biscuits into a food processor and blitz to crumbs. Add the butter and pulse to combine. Tip the mix into a fluted rectangular tart tin, about 10 x 34cm (or 20cm round tin) and press into the base and up the sides right to the edge. Bake for 15 mins until crisp.

STEP 2

While the base is baking, tip the egg yolks, sugar, and lime and lemon zests into a bowl and beat with an electric whisk until doubled in volume. Pour in the condensed milk, beat until combined, then add the citrus juices.

STEP 3

Pour the mix into the tart case and bake for 20 mins until just set with a slight wobble in the centre. Leave to set completely, then remove from the tin, cool and chill. Serve in slices topped with thin lime slices, if you like.

Salted caramel cheesecake

Things Needed

For the base

50g butter, melted, plus extra for the tin

200g chocolate digestives

For the filling and topping

750g (3 tubs) cream cheese

300g caramel sauce (dulce de leche) from a tin or jar

1 tsp vanilla extract

150g golden caster sugar

2 tbsp plain flour

4 medium eggs

Directions

STEP 1

Heat oven to 180C/160C fan/gas 4. Butter a 23cm springform cake tin and line the base with baking parchment. Tip the biscuits into a food processor, blitz to crumbs and pour in the melted butter. (You could also tip the biscuits into a bag, bash with a rolling pin into crumbs and mix in the butter.) Press the biscuit mixture into the base of the tin – the easiest way to do this is by flattening it with your hand under a sheet of cling film. Place the tin on a tray and bake for 10 mins, then remove from the oven to cool.

STEP 2

Meanwhile, scrape the cream cheese into a bowl with 3 tbsp of the caramel sauce, the vanilla, sugar and flour, and beat until smooth. Beat in the eggs, one at a time, until you have a thick, smooth custard consistency. Tip over the base, scraping the bowl clean, and bake in the oven for 10 mins. Reduce the temperature to 140C/120C fan/gas 1 and continue to bake for 25-30 mins until there is a slight wobble in the centre. Turn off the heat and leave the door just slightly ajar – a tea towel holding the door open is ideal. This should leave you with a completely smooth top, but if there are a couple of small cracks, don't worry. Leave the cheesecake in the oven until completely cool (overnight is fine), then chill until needed. Will keep in the fridge for two days.

STEP 3

On the day, loosen the sides of the cheesecake from the tin with a knife and remove the base (although I usually serve it straight from the tin base). Add a large pinch of flaky sea salt to the rest of the caramel sauce, then spoon it over the cake and swirl with the back of the spoon. The cheesecake will sit happily on a stand at room temperature for a couple of hours. Just before serving, sprinkle with extra sea salt, if you like.

Eton mess cheesecake

Things Needed

100g butter, plus extra for the tin

200g digestive biscuits

375g mascarpone

420g full-fat cream cheese

150g icing sugar, plus 2 tbsp for the strawberries

1 vanilla pod, seeds scraped, pod reserved

225ml double cream

600g strawberries, hulled, larger ones cut in half

1 tbsp balsamic vinegar

10 shop-bought mini meringues

edible flowers to decorate (optional)

Directions

STEP 1

Butter a 20cm springform cake tin and line the base with baking parchment. Put the biscuits in a plastic bag and use a rolling pin to bash them into crumbs – or blitz in a food processor. Melt the butter, then stir it into the biscuit crumbs, mixing thoroughly. Tip into the tin, press down to create a firm layer and put in the fridge for 1 hr to set.

STEP 2

Using an electric whisk, beat the cheeses, sugar, vanilla seeds and a pinch of salt until thick and smooth. Pour in the double cream and whisk until only just combined. Spoon the filling onto the base, smooth the top and return to the fridge for at least 4 hrs or overnight.

STEP 3

Half an hour before serving, put the strawberries in a bowl with 2 tbsp icing sugar, the balsamic and scraped vanilla pod. Mix once, then leave the strawberries to soften slightly and release their juices. Push 1/4 of the strawberries through a sieve along with the juices to create a thick purée – or blitz in a food processor.

STEP 4

To serve, run a knife around the outside of the cheesecake, release it from the tin, then top with the strawberries dotted with the meringues, crushing some as you go. Drizzle over the purée and decorate with flowers, if using.

LUPUS-FRIENDLY SNACKS RECIPES

One-pot garlic chicken

Things Needed

4 medium chicken breasts, skin removed, sliced crosswise into thick strips

75g plain flour

2 tbsp olive or rapeseed oil

50g unsalted butter

10-15 small garlic cloves, or to taste

250ml hot chicken stock

100ml double cream

30g Parmigiano-Reggiano, finely grated

small bunch of flat-leaf parsley, finely chopped (optional)

cooked rice and steamed green beans, to serve (optional)

Directions

STEP 1

Tip the chicken into a shallow bowl and sprinkle over the flour. Season well. Heat the oil in a large frying pan over a medium-high heat and fry the chicken, shaking off any excess flour first, for 1-2 mins until lightly golden all over. (You may need to do this in batches.)

STEP 2

Reduce the heat to medium and add the butter. Peel as many garlic cloves as you prefer, and drop these into the pan. Cook for 5 mins until the garlic has turned lightly golden, stirring to keep the chicken from burning.

STEP 3

Pour in the stock and simmer for 10 mins until the garlic is tender. Add the cream and cheese and simmer for a further 5 mins until the sauce thickens slightly. Taste for seasoning and adjust as needed. Scatter with the chopped parsley, if using, and serve hot with rice and green beans, if you like.

White chocolate cheesecake

Things Needed

300g digestive biscuits

150g unsalted butter, melted, plus extra to grease

400g white chocolate, broken into pieces

300g full-fat cream cheese (we used Philadelphia)

250g mascarpone

300ml double cream

200g strawberries or raspberries, to serve

Directions

STEP 1

Crush the biscuits in a food processor until completely ground. Add butter and whizz again until you have the desired crumbly consistency.

STEP 2

Grease and line the base of a 23cm deep, loose-bottomed cake tin. Add the biscuit mixture to the cake tin and pat it flat. Leave to set in the fridge for approximately 30 mins.

STEP 3

Begin melting the chocolate in a heatproof glass bowl over a small pan of hot water on a low heat. Stir occasionally to prevent sticking. Remove from the heat and leave to cool for 10 mins until barely warm but still liquid.

STEP 4

Meanwhile whisk the cream cheese and mascarpone together. Add double cream and keep whisking until the mixture is just holding its own shape. Finally, add the melted chocolate and whisk until just combined.

STEP 5

Spoon the mixture over the cooled and set biscuit base, then smooth the top. Return to the fridge to cool for at least 6 hrs until the topping is set. Finally, decorate with fruit.

Vanilla cupcakes

Things Needed

For the cupcake mixture

120g butter, softened

120g caster sugar

2 egg

1 tsp vanilla extract

120g self-raising flour

For the buttercream icing

140g butter, softened

275g icing sugar

1-2 tbsp milk

A few drops of food colouring (optional)

Directions

STEP 1

Heat oven to 180C/160C fan/gas 4 and line a 12-hole muffin tin with paper cases.

STEP 2

Cream the butter and sugar together in a bowl until pale. Beat the eggs in a separate bowl and mix into the butter mixture along with the vanilla extract.

STEP 3

Fold in the flour, adding a little milk until the mixture is of a dropping consistency. Spoon the mixture into the paper cases until they are three quarters full.

STEP 4

Bake in the oven for 10-15 minutes, or until golden-brown on top and a skewer inserted into one of the cakes comes out clean. Set aside to cool for 5-10 minutes. Then place on a wire rack.

STEP 5

For the buttercream icing, beat the butter until soft. Add half the icing sugar and beat until smooth.

STEP 6

Add the remaining icing sugar with 1 tbsp milk, adding more milk if necessary, until the mixture is smooth and creamy. Add food colouring (optional) and mix well.

STEP 7

Spoon the buttercream into a piping bag and add a nozzle of your choice. Pipe in a swirl motion and then enjoy!

Chocolate brownie cake

Things Needed

100g butter

125g caster sugar

75g light brown or muscovado sugar

125g plain chocolate (plain or milk)

1 tbsp golden syrup

2 eggs

1 tsp vanilla extract/essence

100g plain flour

½ tsp baking powder

2 tbsp cocoa powder

Directions

STEP 1

Heat oven to 180C/fan 160C/gas 4. Grease and line a 20cm cake tin.

STEP 2

Place the butter, caster sugar, brown sugar, chocolate and golden syrup in the pan and melt gently on a low heat until it is smooth and lump-free.

STEP 3

Remove the pan from the heat.

STEP 4

Break the eggs into the bowl and whisk with the fork until light and frothy. 5 Add the eggs, vanilla extract or essence, flour, baking powder and cocoa powder to the chocolate mixture and mix thoroughly.

STEP 5

Put the mixture into the greased and lined cake tin and place on the middle shelf of the oven. Bake for 25-30 mins.

STEP 6

Remove and allow to cool for 20-30 mins before cutting into wedges and serving.

STEP 7

Serve with cream or ice cream and plenty of fresh fruit.

Hearty pasta soup

Things Needed

1 tbsp olive oil

2 carrots, chopped

1 large onion, finely chopped

1l vegetable stock

400g can chopped tomato

200g frozen mixed peas and beans

250g pack fresh filled tortellini (we used spinach and ricotta)

handful of basil leaves (optional)

grated parmesan (or vegetarian alternative), to serve

Directions

STEP 1

Heat oil in a pan. Fry the carrots and onion for 5 mins until starting to soften. Add the stock and tomatoes, then simmer for 10 mins. Add the peas and beans with 5 mins to go.

STEP 2

Once veg is tender, stir in the pasta. Return to the boil and simmer for 2 mins until the pasta is just cooked. Stir in the basil, if using. Season, then serve in bowls topped with a sprinkling of Parmesan and slices of garlic bread.

Red velvet cupcakes

Things Needed

150g plain flour

1 tbsp cocoa powder

1 tsp bicarbonate of soda

50g butter, softened

150g caster sugar

1 large egg, beaten

1 tsp vanilla paste

100ml buttermilk or kefir

50ml vegetable oil

1 tsp white wine vinegar

1 tbsp red gel food colouring

For the cream cheese icing

100g slightly salted butter, softened

225g icing sugar

100g full fat cream cheese, stirred to loosen

Directions

STEP 1

Line a cupcake tin with 12 cupcake cases and set aside. Heat oven to 180C/160C fan/gas 4. Sieve the flour, cocoa, bicarb and a pinch of fine salt into a medium bowl and mix to combine.

STEP 2

Using a stand mixer or an electric hand whisk, beat together the butter and sugar until light and fluffy, then beat in the egg, vanilla, buttermilk, oil and vinegar until combined. Gradually mix the wet Things Neededinto the dried. Once combined, mix in the red food colouring until you have a deep red mix – the colour may vary depending on what brand you use.

STEP 3

Divide the batter between the cupcake cases and bake for 15 mins, or until a skewer inserted into the centre of a cake comes out clean.

STEP 4

While the cakes are cooling, make the icing. Beat together the butter and icing sugar using an electric whisk or by hand until pale and fluffy, about 3 mins, then beat in the cream cheese for a further 1-2 mins until well combined.

STEP 5

Once the cakes are cool, use a piping bag fitted with a star nozzle to cover the cakes with the cream cheese icing, or dollop the icing on top using a spoon.

Dorset apple traybake

Things Needed

225g butter, softened, plus extra for the tin

450g cooking apples (such as Bramley)

½ lemon, juiced

280g golden caster sugar

4 eggs

2 tsp vanilla extract

350g self-raising flour

2 tsp baking powder

demerara sugar, to sprinkle

Directions

STEP 1

Heat the oven to 180C/160C fan/gas 4. Butter and line a rectangular baking tin (approx 27 x 20cm) with baking parchment. Peel, core and thinly slice the apples, then squeeze over the lemon juice. Set aside.

STEP 2

Put the butter, caster sugar, eggs, vanilla, flour and baking powder into a large bowl and mix well until smooth. Spread half the mixture into the prepared tin. Arrange half the apples over the top of the mixture, then repeat the layers. Sprinkle over the demerara sugar.

STEP 3

Bake for 45-50 mins until golden and springy to the touch. Leave to cool for 10 mins, then turn out of the tin and remove the paper. Cut into bars or squares.

Unbelievably easy mince pies

Things Needed

225g cold butter, diced

350g plain flour

100g golden caster sugar

280g mincemeat

1 small egg, beaten

icing sugar, to dust

Directions

STEP 1

To make the pastry, rub the butter into the flour, then mix in the golden caster sugar and a pinch of salt.

STEP 2

Combine the pastry into a ball – don't add liquid – and knead it briefly. The dough will be fairly firm, like shortbread dough. You can use the dough immediately, or chill for later.

STEP 3

Heat the oven to 200C/180C fan/gas 6. Line 18 holes of two 12-hole patty tins, by pressing small walnut-sized balls of pastry into each hole.

STEP 4

Spoon the mincemeat into the pies. Take slightly smaller balls of pastry than before and pat them out between your hands to make round lids, big enough to cover the pies.

STEP 5

Top the pies with their lids, pressing the edges gently together to seal – you don't need to seal them with milk or egg as they will stick on their own. Will keep frozen for up to one month.

STEP 6

Brush the tops of the pies with the beaten egg. Bake for 20 mins until golden. Leave to cool in the tin for 5 mins, then remove to a wire rack. To serve, lightly dust with the icing sugar. Will keep for three to four days in an airtight container.

Apple crumble loaf cake

Things Needed

140g butter, cut into small pieces, plus extra for the tin

250g self-raising flour

2 tsp mixed spice

140g light muscovado sugar

100g raisin

3 large eggs, beaten

2 apples, peeled, cored and chopped

5 tbsp milk

For the topping

1 rounded tbsp plain flour

25g butter

25g light muscovado sugar

1 rounded tbsp roughly chopped hazelnuts

Directions

STEP 1

Heat oven to 160C/140C fan/gas 3. Butter and line the base of a 2-litre loaf tin with baking parchment. Tip the flour and spice into a food processor and add the butter. Whizz to make fine crumbs, then mix in the sugar. Tip into a mixing bowl and stir in the raisins, eggs, apples and milk. Mix well until everything is evenly combined, then spoon into the prepared tin and smooth the top.

STEP 2

To make the topping, rub the flour, butter and sugar through your fingers to make a rough crumble, then stir in the nuts. Sprinkle evenly over the cake mixture and bake for 50-55 mins, until firm to the touch and a fine skewer inserted into the centre comes out clean. Cool in the tin for 15 mins, then turn out and cool on a wire rack.

Halloween pumpkin cake

Things Needed

For the cake

300g self-raising flour

300g light muscovado sugar

3 tsp mixed spice

2 tsp bicarbonate of soda

175g sultanas

½ tsp salt

4 eggs, beaten

200g butter, melted

zest 1 orange

1 tbsp orange juice

500g (peeled weight) pumpkin or butternut squash flesh, grated

For drenching and frosting

200g pack soft cheese

85g butter, softened

100g icing sugar, sifted

zest 1 orange and juice of half

Directions

STEP 1

Heat oven to 180C/fan 160C/gas 4. Butter and line a 30 x 20cm baking or small roasting tin with baking parchment. Put the flour, sugar, spice, bicarbonate of soda, sultanas and salt into a large bowl and stir to combine.

STEP 2

Beat the eggs into the melted butter, stir in the orange zest and juice, then mix with the dry Things Neededtill combined. Stir in the pumpkin. Pour the batter into the tin and bake for 30 minutes, or until golden and springy to the touch.

STEP 3

To make the frosting, beat together the cheese, butter, icing sugar, orange zest and 1 tsp of the juice till smooth and creamy, then set aside in the fridge. When the cake is done, cool for 5 mins then turn it onto a cooling rack. Prick it all over with a skewer and drizzle with the rest of the orange juice while still warm. Leave to cool completely.

STEP 4

If you like, trim the edges of the cake. Give the frosting a quick beat to loosen, then, using a palette knife, spread over the top of the cake in peaks and swirls. If you're making the cake ahead, keep it in the fridge then take out as many pieces as you want 30 mins or so before serving. Will keep, covered, for up to 3 days in the fridge.

CHAPTER 5
CONCLUSION

In closing, the exploration of dietary considerations in the context of lupus management is a journey marked by complexity and nuance, reflective of the multifaceted nature of this autoimmune condition and the diverse experiences of those living with it. As we delve deeper into the intricate interplay between nutrition, inflammation, and immune dysregulation, it becomes increasingly evident that there is no singular, universal approach to dietary intervention for lupus. Instead, individuals are encouraged to embark on a personalized voyage of discovery, guided by principles rooted in scientific understanding, individual needs, and the ever-evolving landscape of research and clinical practice.

Central to this journey is the recognition that diet can serve as both a source of empowerment and a potential therapeutic modality in the management of lupus. By embracing an anti-inflammatory diet rich in nutrient-dense whole foods, individuals may not only mitigate inflammation but also support overall health and well-being. Moreover, the identification and avoidance of potential dietary triggers, such as certain foods or additives, can play a pivotal role in minimizing disease flares and optimizing symptom management.

Yet, amidst the wealth of dietary information and recommendations, it is essential to navigate with discernment and caution, recognizing that what works for one individual may not necessarily be beneficial for another. Factors such as genetics, disease activity, medication use, comorbidities, and personal preferences all contribute to the complexity of dietary decision-making in lupus.

In this spirit, collaboration and communication between individuals with lupus and their healthcare providers are paramount, serving as the cornerstone of effective dietary management. Through open dialogue, shared decision-making, and ongoing monitoring, individuals can cultivate a sense of agency and empowerment in navigating their nutritional journey, informed by evidence-based guidance and personalized insights.

As we look towards the future, the landscape of lupus management continues to evolve, driven by advances in research, clinical practice, and the lived experiences of those affected by the condition. With each step forward, we inch closer towards a deeper understanding of the intricate relationship between diet and lupus, paving the way for innovative approaches to personalized care and holistic well-being.

In the midst of uncertainty and complexity, one thing remains clear: the importance of approaching dietary management in lupus with compassion, curiosity, and resilience. By embracing the journey with an open heart and an open mind, individuals can harness the transformative power of nutrition to foster not only physical health but also emotional well-being and a profound sense of empowerment in the face of lupus.

www.ingramcontent.com/pod-product-compliance
Lightning Source LLC
Chambersburg PA
CBHW051736250726
48659CB00001B/101